Radishes for Natural Healing

Prevention and Curing of Common Ailments through Radishes

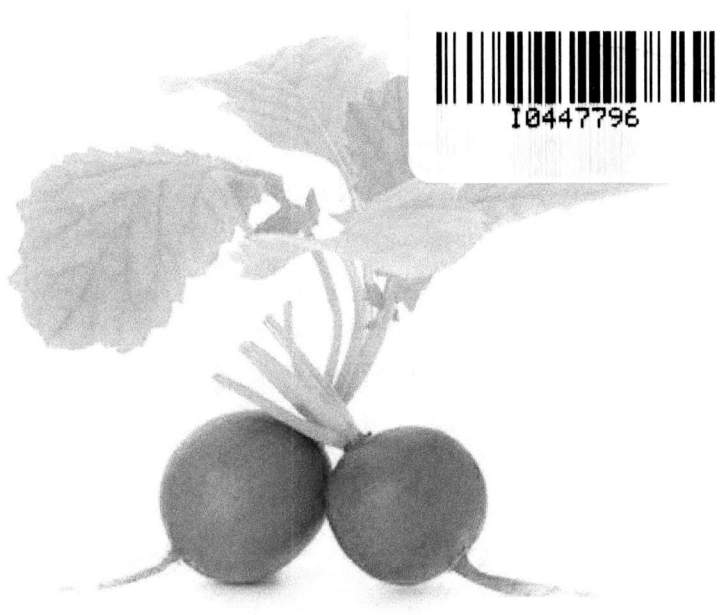

Dueep Jyot Singh

Healthy Learning Series

Mendon Cottage Books

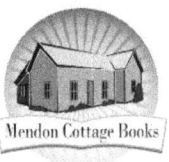

JD-Biz Publishing

Our books are available at

1. Amazon.com
2. Barnes and Noble
3. Itunes
4. Kobo
5. Smashwords
6. Google Play Books

Download Free Books!

http://MendonCottageBooks.com

Table of Contents

Introduction

When I wrote a book upon the magic of radishes a couple of years ago in my" Magic of…" series, I had not known that this vegetable has been used all over the World in order to heal, cure, and prevent a large number of diseases, both common and chronic for millenniums. In that book you learned how to grow radishes and their history, but this book is going to concentrate only about the healing power of radishes, down the ages, along with tips and points about radishes, which you may not know.

The Magic of Radishes - **http://tinyurl.com/j4wsv9x**

Throughout a rather peripatetic life, I have often lived in areas where garlic, onions, and radishes are not eaten very commonly, because some people are very choosy about their strong odor, and for other very finicky people, only commoners/foreigners ate garlic, onions, radishes, and cabbage.

I do not know where and when this particular brand of stupidity started, in culinary circles, and the social acceptance of one of the most healthiest of vegetables available to mankind was banished from normal daily fare because "the best people" did not eat it, and for the majority of the common people out there, it was monkey see monkey do.

But like I said, after having lived in places where onions, garlic, and radishes were not eaten very often in the common diet – that was because I was living in an area where people did not bother about not eating any foods, which were grown underground, including radishes and potatoes, for who knows what ancient traditional, conventional, and possibly religious reasons. I was too young to go into such justifications and explanations, but that meant that anything which was dug up from underneath the ground, was not eaten.

Half of the food items in the World have thus been made taboo or inaccessible to mankind under the label of *forbidden*, with perhaps some justification, or perhaps without any reason or rhyme.

And then, I found myself in another part of the World, where people used to just grab radishes out of the ground, wash them thoroughly to get rid of all the dirt, and then crunch them, without even bothering to peel them. They definitely did not care about flatulence and bad odor in the mouth or any other supposed side effect of eating radishes. Their breakfasts were full of cooked radishes either as a vegetable, or stuffed into bread pancakes, with radishes, onions, and tomato salads to be served with every meal.

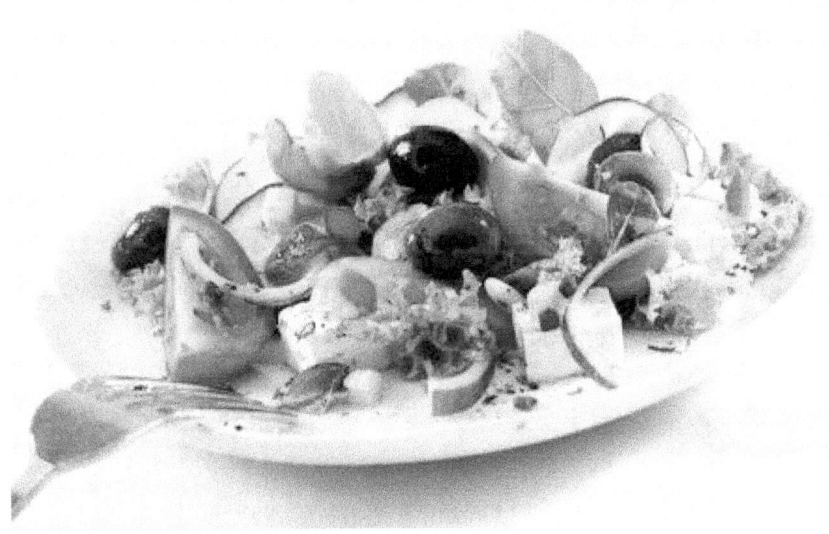

And what I noticed is that these people had really healthy and glowing skin, excellent teeth, plenty of energy, and so much enthusiasm, joie de vivre, and just plain zest for life that I could not keep up with all the physical and mental antics and capers they thought up throughout the day.

Could it have something to do with their diet? And that is why I began to concentrate on that food item which I had been missing/eaten very rarely for the first six years of my life – radishes – and I soon found out that yes, it was radishes that were responsible for their lack of disease and good health.

This tuber can be eaten raw, or in its cooked state. Apart from having been a major part of ancient diets, all over the World, it was also used as a medicine to heal and cure a number of ailments in ancient medical sciences. Korean, Japanese, Egyptian, Greek, Indian, Persian, and other ancient civilizations used either the radish or the juice of a fresh radish to administer to the patient and get rid of any sort of infection or accumulated toxins.

Every single part of the radish is put into use. Radish seeds are diuretics. The leaves can be turned into juice and drank down every day, to keep your skin unblemished and your body toxin free. Just a couple of days ago, I cooked the leaves for lunch and had another new taste added to my repertoire of unusual tastes – cooked radish leaves. You are not going to eat these radishes, either leaves, or in a salad, at night, because there is a chance that you may suffer from joint aches.

I am giving you my experience; I had those radish leaves for dinner, three days ago, even though I was told not to eat them at night. Perhaps that is autosuggestion, but last night I had some pain for the first time in my life, in my small of my back. It could either be lying on my back, instead of curled up on my side, while sleeping to keep my spinal cord limber and so I woke up with stiff muscles and backache. Or it could have been the radishes! However, why take a chance?

Nevertheless, this book is going to tell you all about the benefit of radishes, to keep you healthy throughout your life and especially in the summer.

People eating radishes along with their seeds are never going to suffer from any sort of stones, in their kidneys or in their gallbladder. You can also get oil, from the seeds, which has the radish taste in it. Wonder why nobody thought about using that oil for cooking – radish flavored foods – but possibly it must have been too much of a problem collecting all those seeds, and then extracting that oil.

Just take the leaves of a radish and chew on them like you would do salad leaves. They are prickly, but they have a mild taste. You may also want to chop them up finally and mix them up with other salad greens for a distinctive pungent flavor.

The fruit of the radishes are eaten throughout the World either as a vegetable, cooked, or you can just mix them up, chopped in salads or in yogurt as a dip. You can even take a radish – just scrub it, but do not peel it because most of its nutritive value is under its skin, chop it into pieces, and eat it raw with salt-and-pepper, grate it, or cook it – but whichever way, you eat it, it is going to keep you healthy, it is tasty, and it is good for fighting infections.

According to ancient medical sciences, the radish was essentially a blood purifier. And that is why it was used extensively to cure any sort of problems, especially those faced by adolescents in their growing stage. Skin diseases, especially pimples, and other age-related skin problems were cured with traditional medicines made of radishes, because the idea was that a flawless skin could only be obtained through a clean internal system, which included the blood.

For those who want the scientific explanation of this, radishes have a large amount of iron in them. Anybody eating lots of radishes would never suffer from an iron deficiency, especially when he was a teenager. Also, he would not have any toxins buildup in his system. And that is why this would reflect in his skin, keeping it glowing and fair.

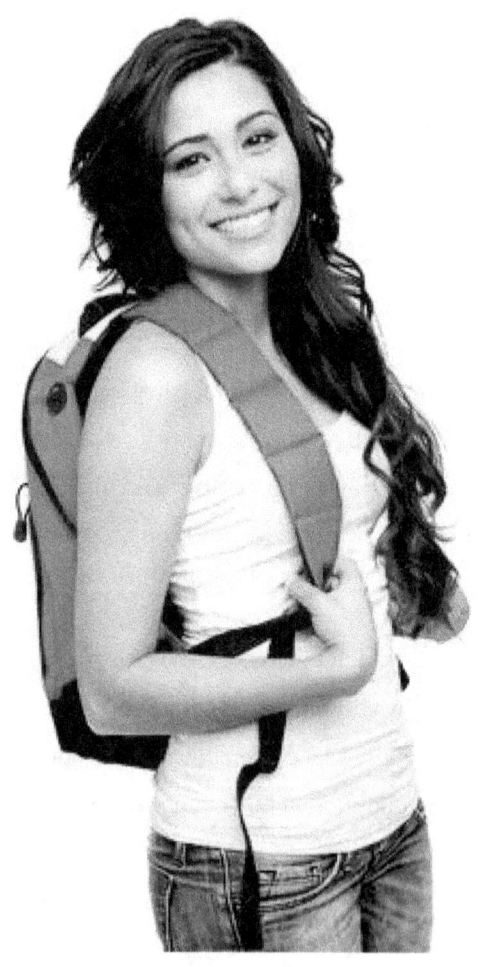

When I was young, a large number of my college mates, both male and female, used to have a tablespoonful of a natural ancient medicine, coming down from Persian medicine called literally – *cleaner*. Its main ingredient was radishes along with other herbs. They had been put on this natural medicine, by their parents when they were 15 so that the blood could be cleansed, and also because every parent wanted their child to have unblemished, glowing, soft and silky, very attractive healthy skin.

Even though a radish is not very mild, when you taste it – it is rather pungent – the taste can be accentuated with salt, pepper, and lemon juice. You may also want to eat it without any sort of spice addition, fresh from the garden and washed under the garden tap.

Radishes are considered to be very good for the eyes and teeth. In many parts of the World, children are given radishes to chew, not only to get a strong dental set, but also to polish their teeth naturally, and get rid of all that extra plaque buildup.

In ancient medicine, radishes have been known to get rid of bile diseases, chest infections, and digestion related diseases. They are also used to prevent fever, eye infections, nose infections, throat infections, and gallbladder problems. Radish leaves are excellent for your stomach, because apart from being salad greens, they prevent constipation and promote healthy hunger.

In ancient times, radish leaves were considered to be more nourishing, along with its juice, and that is why whenever I see anybody throwing radish leaves away, because for them, it is something prickly and not so important, I say to myself, oh boy, what a waste. These leaves are easily digested, especially if you eat them throughout the year, but not in the winter, without the accompaniment of other vegetables like tomatoes or carrots.

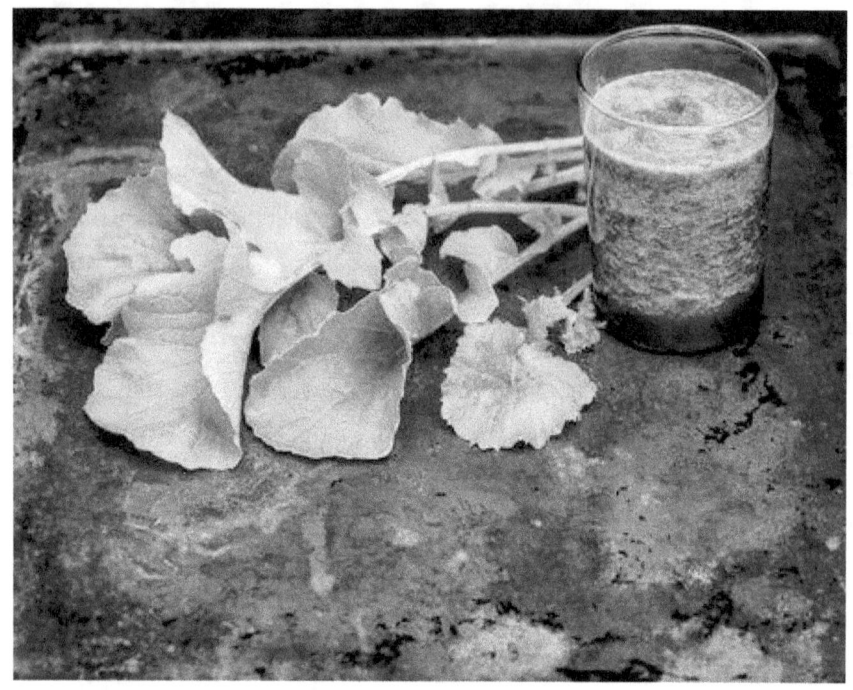

Do not eat the leaves raw; cook them before you eat them. That is because raw leaves may cause possible problems in your gallbladder. Also smaller radishes – half grown radishes – are more easily digestible than fully grown totally ripe radishes.

The larger the radishes are they are going to be more "rich, dry, hot in Constitution and promoters of the fundamental constitutional bio – elements – air, fire, and water." This is, of course, in Ayurvedic medicine, when all the bio elements have to be in harmony for good health and if any food item encourages or promotes any of these bio elements making up the Constitution of a normal human being, he is going to fall sick.

These are the ancient medical theories, on which alternative medicine has relied, down the ages. That is why those medical practitioners knew how to balance these bio elements for continual good health through proper diet.

And I think that is the reason why radishes are never eaten on an empty stomach. This is going to cause heartburn and acidity. Again, this is not a winter food, when eaten on its own, even though many people keep eating it throughout the year, and then wonder why they suffer from joint pain in the winter.

Radish seeds are normally used as appetite promoters. You can also grind them up and use them as a spice. In ancient times, they were boiled in water, and this water drunk to get rid of gallstones and kidney stones. Sore throats can be cured by grinding the seeds, mixing them with hot water and drinking down this concoction. Also, skin diseases can be cured permanently by just making up a ground mixture of radish seeds with lemon juice and applied on eczema, skin infections, and other external skin ailments.

Radish juice is excellent for urinary infections, piles, and for controlling diabetes. Just grind the small variety of radishes and drink their juice down, early in the morning. They are going to help cure chronic ailments, and keep your skin toxin free. We are so used to eating those large overripe radishes, that when we find ourselves feeling "not too good," we do not know that it is the powerful radish which is acting on our digestive system. The smaller variety and a smaller sized radish is equally powerful, but it does not have a longer lasting after effect on your digestive system!

Use the green and soft new leaves of the radishes. It is much more preferable to eat them cooked, even though a couple of radish leaves can be chopped up finely and added to other salad greens like cabbages, spinach, and other leaves.

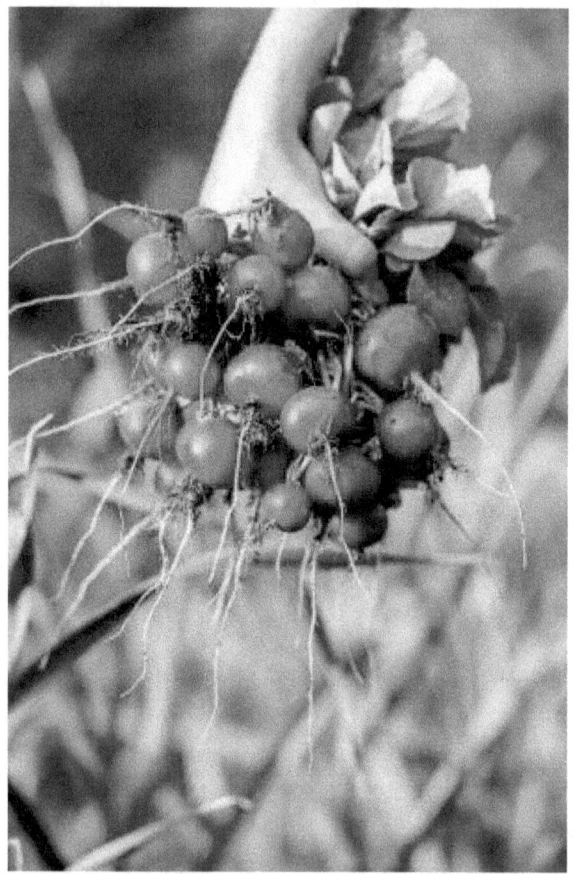

When you are cooking the leaves, do not use too much salt for flavoring because that is going to counteract the beneficial power of the leaves. On the other hand, cooking, radishes and eating them is going to destroy its nutritional proteins and minerals. So you should eat them raw.

The leaves are capable of cleaning your system and getting rid of infections in the digestive and urinary system. The radish root has been known to cure and prevent piles, jaundice, and skin diseases like vitiligo. Radish seeds were ground to a paste in water and used by the ancient Greeks and Romans to prevent skin blemishes and get rid of wrinkles.

The radishes you can get worldwide can be anywhere from 10 cm to 25 cm in length, depending on the varieties and species and even more. They are either going to be white in color or red or small white. The white species is more prevalent than red radishes.

Apart from the iron, calcium, and sodium content present in radishes, the fat content is 0.1% and the protein content is 0.7%, 94.4% of radish content is water. Along with that, radishes also have vitamin C, vitamin B complex, and phosphorus in them.

You are not going to eat radishes if you suffer from ulcers or acidity.

Radishes to Cure Stomach Ailments

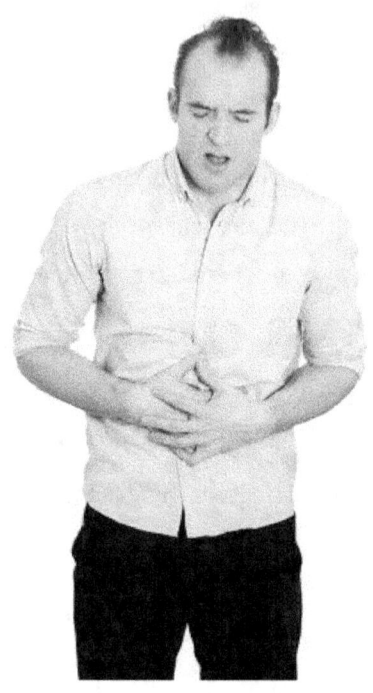

There are a number of common stomach ailments which have been the bane of mankind since time began. It could either be because of a change in diet or possibly due to overeating. These ailments include indigestion, flatulence, dyspepsia, loss of appetite, constipation, diarrhea, heartburn, dropsy, ulcers, and acidity.

Radishes are going to prevent, as well as cure, all these ailments.

Indigestion

Indigestion is one of the most common of stomach ailments, and is caused due to eating all sorts of foods and at odd hours, eating too much rich and spicy fare, over stuffing yourself just because you could not resist all the delicious food, right in front of you and so your stomach suddenly decides to give in.

It is going to stop digesting everything in a natural manner, and stop working at one hundred percent efficiency. And the result is going to be that all the food which was digested properly before is going to sit in the stomach, being digested at a milder and slower pace.

This food which should have been eliminated in the natural manner, hours ago, is now going to stay in your stomach and digestive system producing toxic poisons. So to prevent indigestion, you are going to take a radish and cut it lengthwise. You are going to take the juice of one lemon and some rock salt/black salt and sprinkle it in the cut. Now chew this so that the saliva assimilates the radish as well as the lemon. You can also take two – four green young leaves of the radish along with it.

Remember to eat one radish as a salad for lunch. You are going to have a light meal at night. And you are never going to suffer from indigestion again.

Dyspepsia

Dyspepsia is normally caused when your digestive system is not working properly, and the system is constipated. That means the half digested food is not eliminated naturally. You need to get rid of dyspepsia as fast as possible because it can give rise to a large number of other problems.

Stop eating rich and spicy foods, as well as fried foods, immediately. Try eating light meals, including salads, or try fasting for one day, when you are not going to eat anything solid, but drinking fresh fruit juice and eat raw vegetables and fresh fruit. This is going to give your digestive system a little bit of respite. It is also not going to overtax its digestive capacities.

DYSPEPSIA

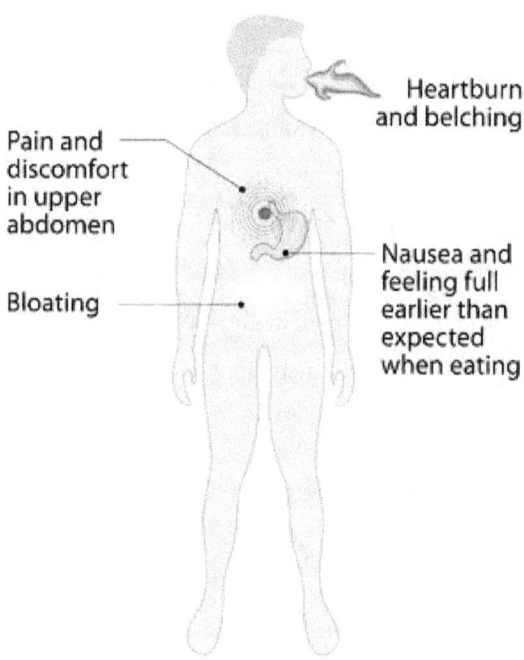

Pain and discomfort in upper abdomen

Heartburn and belching

Bloating

Nausea and feeling full earlier than expected when eating

The curing is going to be done by taking 200 mL of radish juice. To this, you are going to add 50 grams of bishops weed and 10 g of rock salt. Why did I not add sea salt, you may ask? That is because rock salt is normally found in its pure form in solid chunks of rock, which you are going to grind right in your kitchen. But the sea salt which you are going to buy from your supermarket shelf has been defined, preservatives added to it, it has been iodized and all sorts of modern-day additives have been added supposedly to make the sea salt more effective and beneficial.

The real nutritional food value of the sea salt has thus been leached away in the refining process. So that is the reason why I always suggest rock salt or black salt, whenever I am making anything to cure myself or advising my friends. This is salt in its purest form. It is also full of minerals and natural goodness.

This mixture is now going to be put out in the shade so that the seeds can soak up the goodness of the radish juice, after you have squeezed the juice of three lemons on it. The radish and the lemon juice combination are going to make sure that you never suffer from any stomach ailments ever again. Drying in the shade means drying in the open air, in a covered utensil, under a tree or in one corner of your airy and sunny porch/terrace/balcony.

It is going to take about 10 – 12 days for this juice to be absorbed in the seeds, through this sunshade drying.

The moment all the liquid power has been absorbed into the seeds, you are going to grind it and put it into in an airtight bottle. The moment you find yourself suffering from any sort of dyspepsia, you are going to take just one pinch twice a day. By the next day you are going to find your dyspepsia a thing of the past.

A number of people have asked me why I am so careful about the amount of natural remedies to be taken – like one pinch/half a teaspoon/and no more and no less. That is because this is the amount which is needed by Mother Nature to cure you. But human beings being human beings think that more is always better. That means when I say one pinch, they had better take two pinches, because that will make the medicine more powerful and more efficient and also give a faster result, isn't it so?

Nature's logic does not work that way. And down the ages, people have got to know all about the quantities of natural curative ingredients, needed to keep one healthy. So that is why one pinch! One pinch twice a day means two pinches throughout the day.

Flatulence

People suffering from indigestion and dyspepsia are going to suffer from flatulence because the food which is still in its indigested state has not been eliminated from the system naturally. And so the undigested food starts rotting in the stomach, emitting "gases."

You are going to cure flatulence with 125 g of radish juice with 125 mL of carrot juice. This is going to expel the accumulated gases and also get rid of the bloating. You can also take a mixture of radishes and tomato juice to get rid of the flatulence.

Constipation

Constipation is also one of the most common stomach ailments known to man. This is normally caused through eating rich and spicy food, indigestion, and other digestion related problems.

The constipation cure is the same as the indigestion cure by taking pieces of radish with lemon juice and black salt; along with four – five green leaves. If the constipation is chronic, you are going to take the powder, of which I gave you the recipe a couple of pages above. You are going to take this pinch, before going to sleep at night, with hot water.

Diarrhea

Diarrhea is a symptom of any sort of infection which prevents your food from being digested properly. Under such circumstances, the infection causes the bowels to be eliminated in a liquid form instead of a solid fecal form. You may also find pieces of the inner stomach lining, appearing with the diarrhea flow and in serious cases, you can also see blood in the excreted matter.

Naturally, any sort of blood appearing anywhere without a justified reason needs an immediate medical checkup, but if the diarrhea is just what is called "loose motions," it can be for a number of other reasons too, including a change in the weather and temperature outside, or perhaps eating something which has disagreed with your system and the system getting rid of it more quickly.

You may also suffer from stomach cramps, if the diarrhea is acute. The patient is going to get dehydrated because the valuable nutrients of his body are being eliminated really fast, in the stools. That is why the patients are given a natural oral rehydration solution of water with salt and sugar mixed in it. This balances the salt content in the body, a depletion of which can cause acute dehydration in the patient.

Radishes are extremely efficient in stopping diarrhea. But for this, you are going to make a radish soup/decoction with radish and water and give it to the patient.

Chop up a radish into small pieces and put 4 cups of water in the vessel. Put on to boil. Add some ginger and some salt. When the water has been reduced to just one cup, give it to the patient after filtering the radish tea.

Prepare this fresh, three – four times a day depending on how severe the attack of diarrhea is. The patient is going to be cured by the next morning.

Stomachache

A pain in the stomach can be due to a number of reasons - either having hurt your stomach internally and inadvertently, or possibly due to some infection in the stomach region.

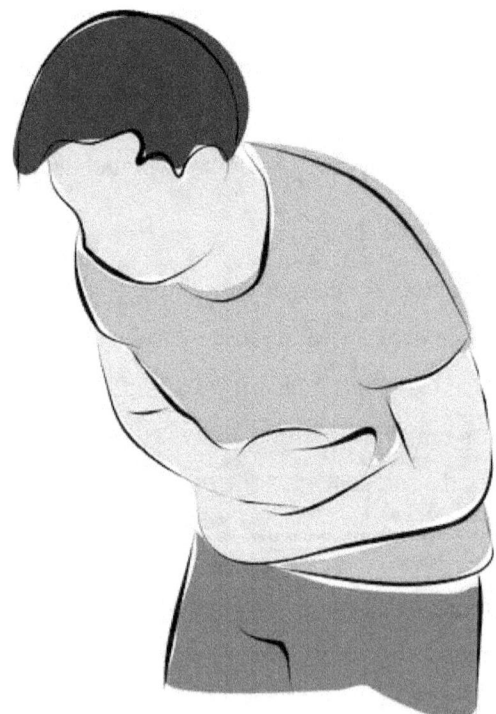

For this, a little bit of radish is going to help cure any problem. Take a small raw radish. Take the juice of one lemon and sprinkle it all over the radish. Then take a number of mint leaves, grind them up together and spread them all over this radish lemon salad. You are going to have it for lunch because you do not eat radishes on an empty stomach.

This is going to heal any sort of stomachache brought about through an infection or any other possible problem in your stomach.

Dropsy

Any sort of swelling in the body, which we call edema today was once called dropsy when it occurred in the stomach. It is also called ascites.

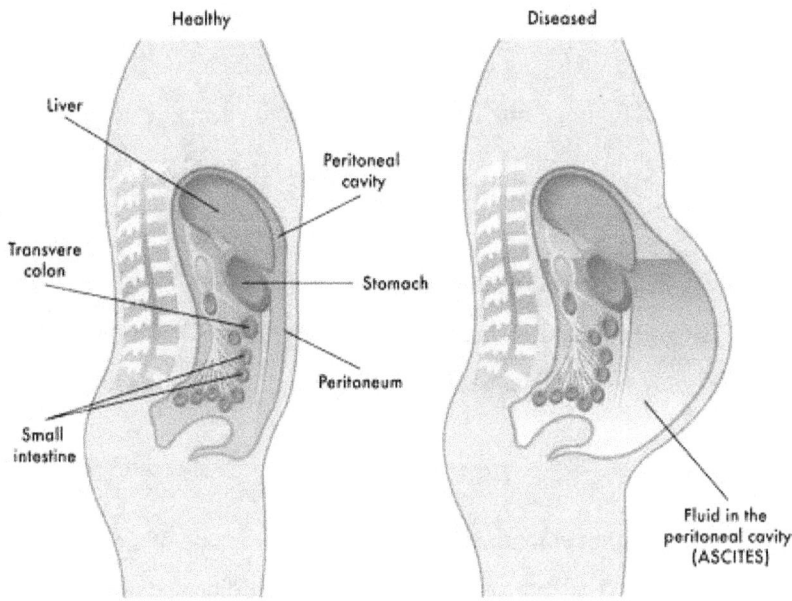

Edema can be a symptom of a number of problems in your body, and you may find your hands and feet swelling up. But when you find a swelling in your stomach region that is the sign of dropsy.

This swelling is made up of water collecting in the stomach region. So when you lie down and turn on your side, the water also shifts to that same side and this is going to cause you a lot of discomfort. Your stomach is going to swell up and you are going to feel really lethargic.

Dropsy is cured with fresh radish juice.

You are going to take just 10 g of radish juice (2 teaspoons) to which you are going to add the fresh juice from a gingerroot. Mix the ginger and the radish together, and you are going to feed the patient just **one teaspoonful** of this mixture. Do this thrice a day. All the accumulated water is going to pass out of the patient's system within the next two – three days. The swelling is going to go away and the patient is going to feel immediate relief. So the next time your doctor hands you a diuretic which he says is going to be helpful in getting rid of the dropsy and edema, just say thank you and no, politely, come home, get out your radish and your ginger and heal yourself naturally.

Naturally, when you are healing yourself with radish and ginger for dropsy you are not going to take even one teeny-weeny bit of salt. Salt helps in the retention of the water in the body instead of helping to eliminate it.

Flatulence

Flatulence is a rather embarrassing problem symptomatic of a change in lifestyle and diet. That is because food does not get digested properly and naturally. Along with that, we have the bad habit of eating everything upon which we can lay our hands whenever we want to eat, without bothering about the effect it can have on our digestive systems.

Also with the passing of time, there is going to be a change in the strength of our digestive system. What we could manage to digest in our 20s and 30s is going to be a bit difficult to digest in our 60s and 70s. Also, flatulence has a number of disagreeable side effects including one feeling lazy and lethargic and possibly also feeling pain in the limbs.

Here is how you are going to get rid of flatulence with a radish salad with some fresh leaves added. Add some pieces of cucumber. Now sprinkle some rock salt on this salad, with some lemon juice. This is going to get rid of all the flatulence.

You can also try out radish juice to get rid of flatulence. Do not peel the radish when you are juicing it. You can also grate the radish, and drink the juice. Do not add any salt to this juice. Do not peel the cucumber either. It is going to take a little while – up to 15 to 20 days in chronic cases of flatulence to heal you – but the long-term effects are worthwhile.

Ulcers

Like any part of your body, there is a chance that the tissue in the stomach can also get injured due to the effect of something toxic or harmful. When this happens in the intestines or in the stomach region, you are given pills by your doctor. These pills are not going to cure the ulcers but are going to mask the symptoms so that you think that they have been cured.

You are going to cure yourself with radishes, either as a salad, chopped up in pieces and eaten with tomatoes, or cut lengthwise with the juice of a lemon sprinkled on it. The green leaves of radishes also have to be eaten to make the cure more permanent and effective. While the ulcers are being cured, do not eat anything indigestible, full of proteins, rich and spicy, but have a light diet of fruit, vegetables, and juices.

Acidity/Acid Reflux

Have you found yourself regurgitating something sour and full of bile, some hours after a very rich and spicy meal? This normally occurs when the stomach is trying to digest some spicy, rich, fatty, proteinaceous, or sour food item. The acidic nature of the food is going to attack the stomach and the stomach lining, and you are going to suffer from acidity.

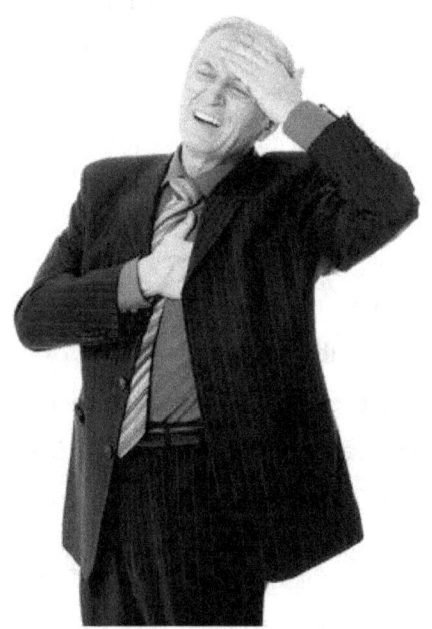

Heartburn/acidity/acid reflux can attack anyone, anytime, anywhere. And it can leave you feeling headachy.

Apart from literally leaving a sour taste in your mouth, you may find yourself suffering from discomfort in your stomach and chest region which you may know as heartburn. You may also belch a bit too often and that leaves a sour sensation/taste in the back of your throat.

This acidity is also going to have a harmful effect upon your liver. You may also suffer from acidity, if you are suffering from calcium deprivation.

This is going to be cured with radishes which you are going to add to your daily diet. Try eating one radish on which you have sprinkled the juice of one lemon, every morning and take a salad of tomatoes, carrots, and radishes regularly for lunch. To get rid of chronic acidity, drink the juice of half a radish.

Someone asked me what I did with the grated radish, which was left over after I had juiced it. I said that it was delicious as a cooked vegetable or if I had some portion of my body swelling up due to any reason, I would just apply the paste on to that region to have that swelling go way down and fast.

You can also use the radish pith upon skin infections, especially eczema or hives.

Radishes to Cure Chronic Diseases

Apart from the stomach ailments which can be cured with the regular intake of radishes as salads, raw green radish leaves, and radish juice, radishes have also been known to cure a number of chronic diseases.

Radishes for Your Heart

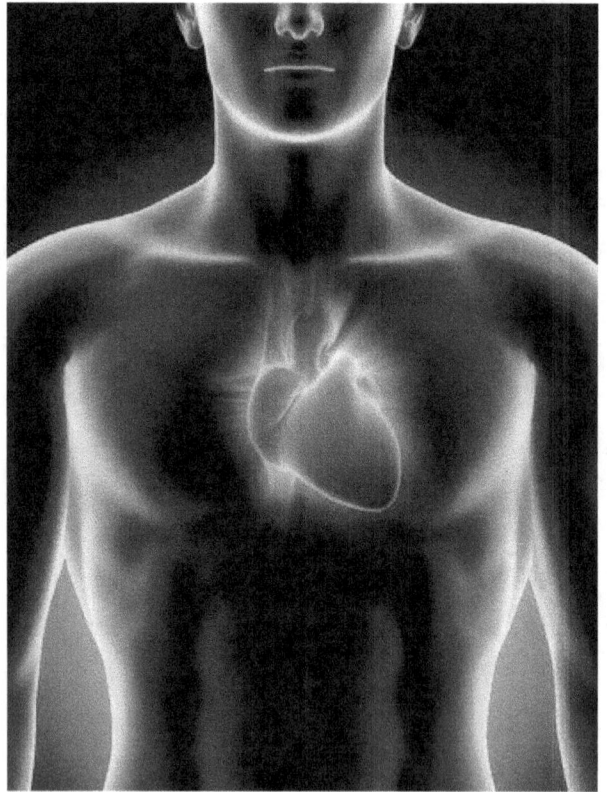

If you are leading a sedentary lifestyle, you may find yourself suffering from some heart problems and ailments later on in your life. Also stress, strain, and tension, especially in today's rat race is capable of having an adverse effect on your heart. But radishes are capable of preventing the buildup of cholesterol in your arteries. Thanks to their potassium content, you are not going to have a weak heart ever.

If you think that there is the possibility of you ever suffering from heart disease or a problem, potentially in the future, because you are genetically inclined to it, start drinking radish juice every day. Also eat at least one fresh radish with your meals. No wonder the oldies that lived up to the 80s and 90s in olden times, always had a salad of onions and radishes for lunch, along with their meals.

Jaundice

Jaundice occurs when the red blood corpuscles in your body do not get eliminated in the normal manner, but creates a product named Bilirubin in your body instead. This gives your skin a yellow tinge. It also leaves the whites of your eyes with a yellow tint.

Jaundice is a symptom of a problem in your kidneys and the best cure for it is radishes. Take 200 mL of radish juice from the leaves. Now add 2 teaspoons full of rock candy to this juice, and drink it every day. You will need 200 mL once a day, for about seven – eight days. This is enough to help cure your jaundice.

This is the only time when you are going to be eating radishes on an empty stomach, early in the morning. You can also take one radish eaten unsalted and raw and 125 mL of radish juice with rock candy. If you add a little bit of sugar cane juice – if available – to this radish juice, you are going to have the healing power of sugarcane working for you too.

For lunch you are going to have a salad of radishes, tomatoes, and chopped apples.

Diabetes

Did you know that it is very easy to control diabetes, as well as even cure it, with radishes? Nobody is going to spend billions of dollars in researching this particular timeworn remedy because there is going to be ample proof that this has been done and can be done, and then how is the allopathic medical association, which is based on science, suppose to sell their expensive drugs supposedly used for controlling diabetes?

If you have somebody in the family suffering from diabetes, and who wants to get away from the side effects of these powerful drugs, this is what you are going to do. Take the fresh leaves of radishes and cook them without any spices or salt. You can either broil them or boil them, as long as they are cooked. Feed them to the patient for lunch. You are going to see the visible positive affect of the leaves' healing qualities within the month. Do not stop this treatment *until the diabetes is cured permanently.*

This means depending on the severity of the state or its chronic nature, the leaves are capable of curing a diabetes patient. Also give him plenty of radish juice obtained from a small fresh radish, every day. The sodium content is going to benefit the patient positively.

High and Low Blood Pressure

Low and high blood pressure is a common ailment in a large number of us, especially when we suffer from stress and tension. If you are suffering from low blood pressure, just take some radish juice, half a glassful is enough – add some rock salt to it and drink it down. The sodium in the salt is going to raise your blood pressure. The radish is going to steady your system.

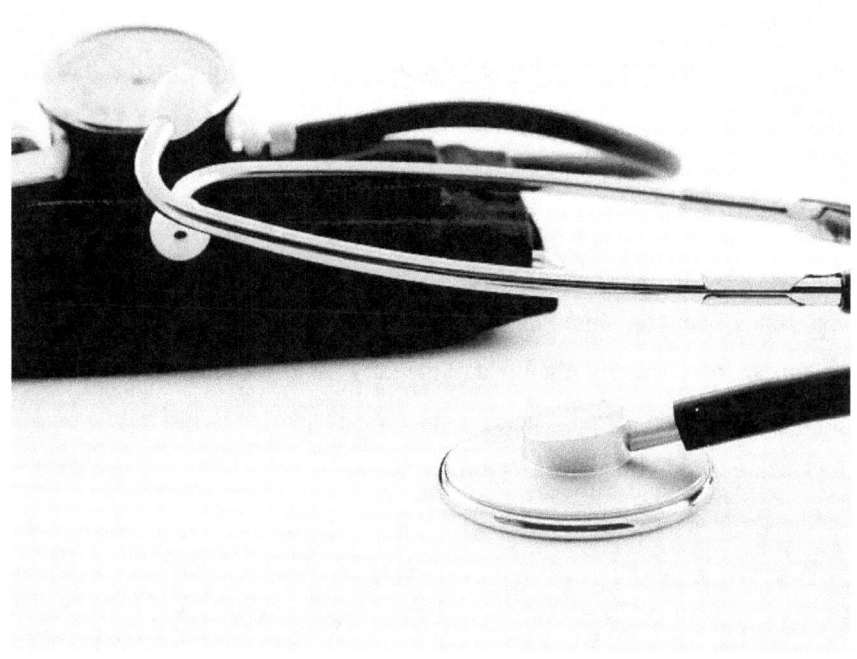

You can also take the powder of dried radishes – chop them up in pieces, and sun dry them – half a teaspoon with 2 teaspoons full of honey once a day. In olden times, this was used to cure ailments in the blood and also to prevent anemia. And if you have spinach leaves around, mix them up with radish leaves, juice them, and drink the juice. Consider that to be your breakfast smoothie every day, and you are going to be surprised at the change in your blood pressure, health, and even skin.

Do not drink more than one glassful of radish juice in a day. If any remedy calls for drinking radish juice, two – three times a day, regulate the quantities so that you manage just one glassful throughout the day.

For high blood pressure, remember that if you have been eating radishes in salads for lunch every day, there is no question of you suffering from high blood pressure ever, however much you are stressed, strained, or are full of tension! But this salad is going to be without any lemon juice and salt. You can instead substitute tomatoes and cucumbers in the salad.

Weight loss

This is one remedy where we are going to be drinking radish juice three – four times a day, but not more than 60 mL throughout the day. This is a long-term treatment but it gets rid of the fatty tissue slowly and steadily. Try drinking this fresh juice of radishes and radish leaves with just a little bit of rock salt added to it at intervals of four hours.

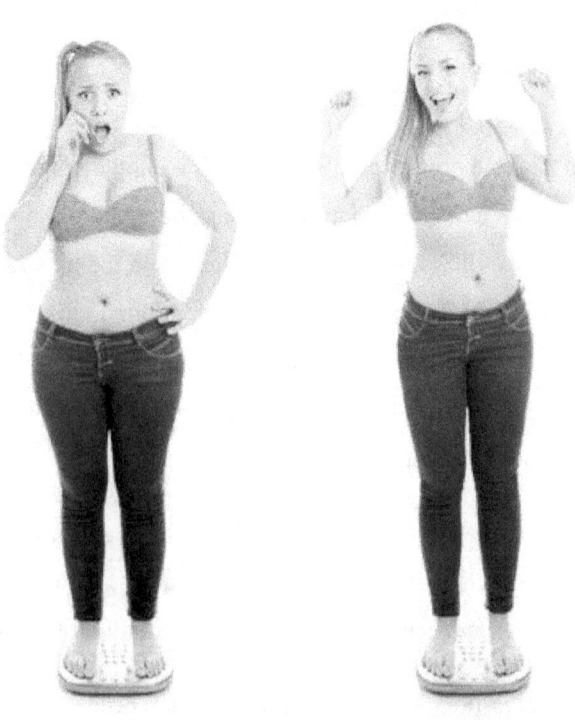

Do not stop this treatment midway, just because you do not get the results overnight. The human body does not lose weight overnight unless one is drastically sick. And many of us think that we do not have all the time in the World to wait patiently for some treatment to work because we cannot see visible results right now.

Mother Nature does not work that way. So let the radishes and the juice get rid of the toxin buildup, which is possibly a part of your cellulite tissue, and allow the fat to melt away as naturally as possible.

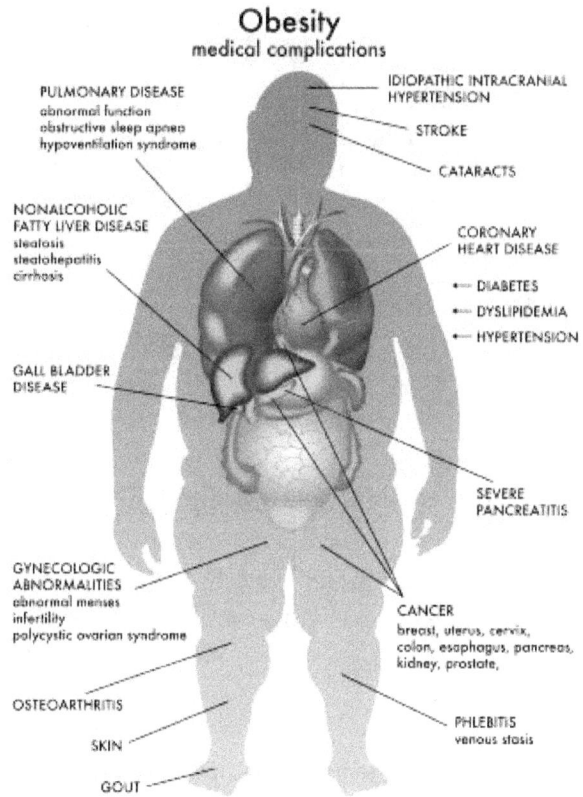

Problems caused due to obesity, the results are worth it

Gout

Gout is normally caused when uric acid crystals build up in the joints, leading to a painful case of arthritis. Again, you are going to be drinking lots of radish juice, 50 – 60 mL throughout the day, but this is going to be a combination of ginger juice and cabbage juice to make up the quantity. Try it out if you are suffering from gout.

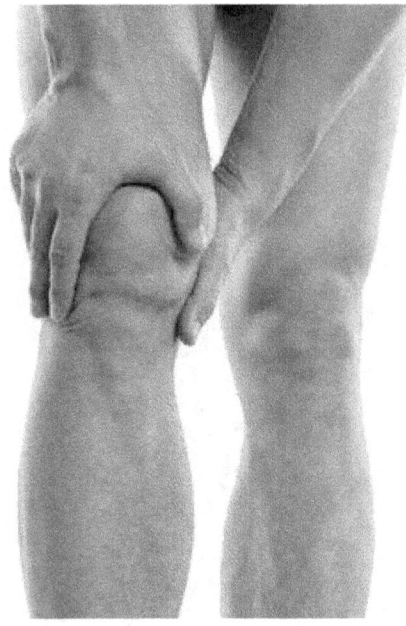

Joint pain and inflammation can be prevented and cured with radish juice.

You may want to crush some radish seeds and apply the paste in a massage procedure all over the painful and inflamed joints and areas. The paste is made traditionally by grinding the radish seeds, and then heating them slowly in sesame oil. Massage the inflamed areas with the oil and apply the seeds on the joints. Bandage with a piece of clean cotton bandage so that the oil and the seeds can do their magic work. You are going to see the magical effect of this, even in chronic arthritis cases, where the patient was not able to move about, in just two weeks.

Conclusion

This book has just giving you some curative properties of radishes, and I have just touched the tip of the iceberg. Radishes can also cure skin diseases and respiratory problems. However, many of the remedies which I have given here are capable of curing infections naturally and permanently, and you may find any skin condition or infection, improving with the application of a little bit of radish pith or even radish juice.

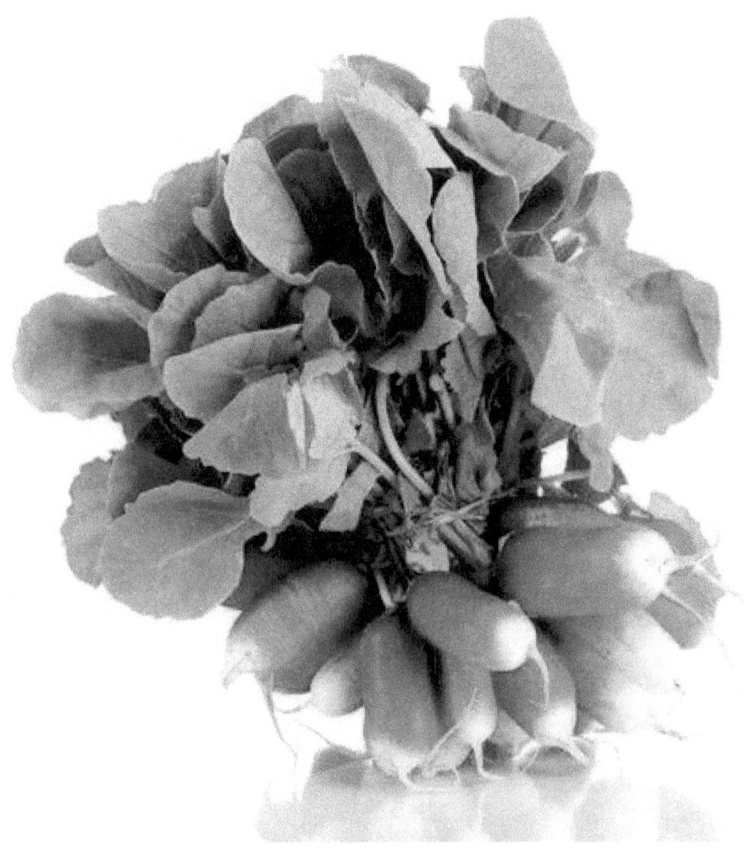

So remember that nature is the best healer and her remedies are powerful enough to cure one or all the ailments, brought about by unhealthy lifestyles, including diet and stress. So put faith in her healing capacities, and have patience. That is because nothing can be cured overnight. The body has to get back into its state of natural health and that can only be done slowly and steadily through natural curing.

Major chronic illnesses can take anywhere between 3 to 6 months to get cured permanently. Small ailments can take anywhere between 2 to 4 days or even less, depending on the virulence of the infection or disease.

So next time you are in the garden, just take out a young radish, wash it, and before anybody can say *what's up Doc,* start chewing like Bugs Bunny. It is good for your teeth, good for your health, and best of all, you are eating something totally fresh and organic.

Live Long and Prosper!

Author Bio

Dueep Jyot Singh is a Management and IT Professional who managed to gather Postgraduate qualifications in Management and English and Degrees in Science, French and Education while pursuing different enjoyable career options like being an hospital administrator, IT,SEO and HRD Database Manager/ trainer, movie , radio and TV scriptwriter, theatre artiste and public speaker, lecturer in French, Marketing and Advertising, ex-Editor of Hearts On Fire (now known as Solstice) Books Missouri USA, advice columnist and cartoonist, publisher and Aviation School trainer, ex-moderator on Medico.in, banker, student councilor ,travelogue writer … among other things!

One fine morning, she decided that she had enough of killing herself by Degrees and went back to her first love—writing. It's more enjoyable! She already has 48 published academic and 14 fiction- in- different- genre books under her belt.

When she is not designing websites or making Graphic design illustrations for clients , she is browsing through old bookshops hunting for treasures, of which she has an enviable collection – including R.L. Stevenson, O.Henry, Dornford Yates, Maurice Walsh, De Maupassant, Victor Hugo, Sapper, C.N. Williamson, "Bartimeus" and the crown of her collection- Dickens "The Old Curiosity Shop," and "Martin Chuzzlewit" and so on… Just call her "Renaissance Woman" - collecting herbal remedies, acting like Universal Helping Hand/Agony Aunt, or escaping to her dear mountains for a bit of exploring, collecting herbs and plants, and trekking.

Check out some of the other JD-Biz Publishing books

Gardening Series on Amazon

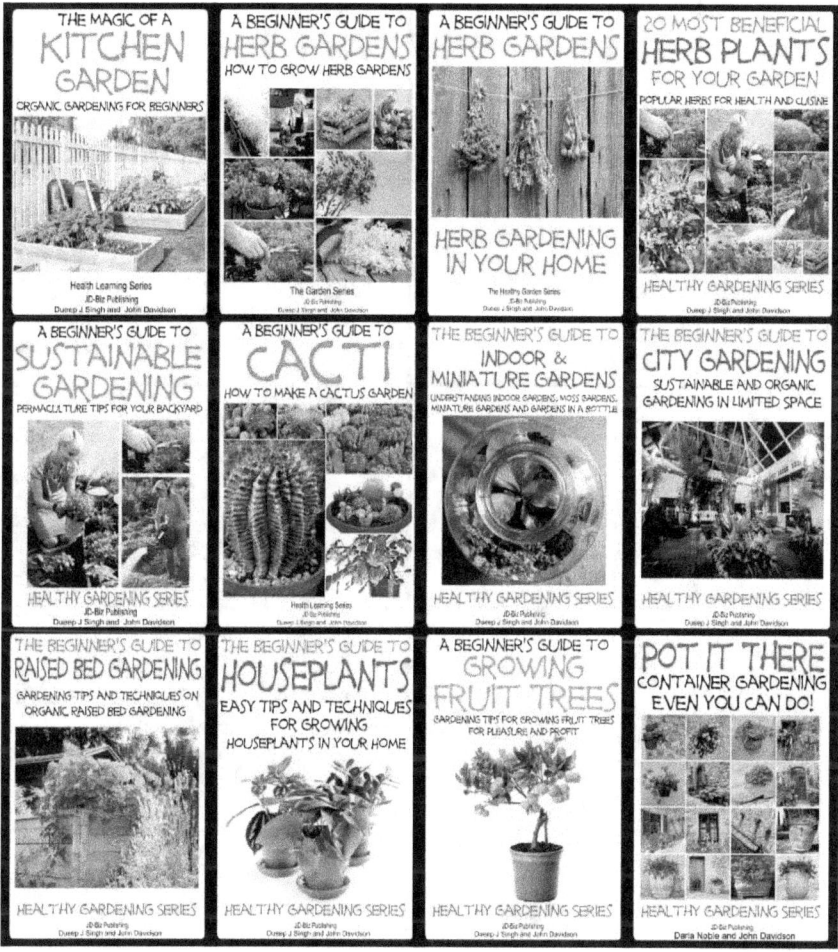

Download Free Books!

http://MendonCottageBooks.com

Health Learning Series

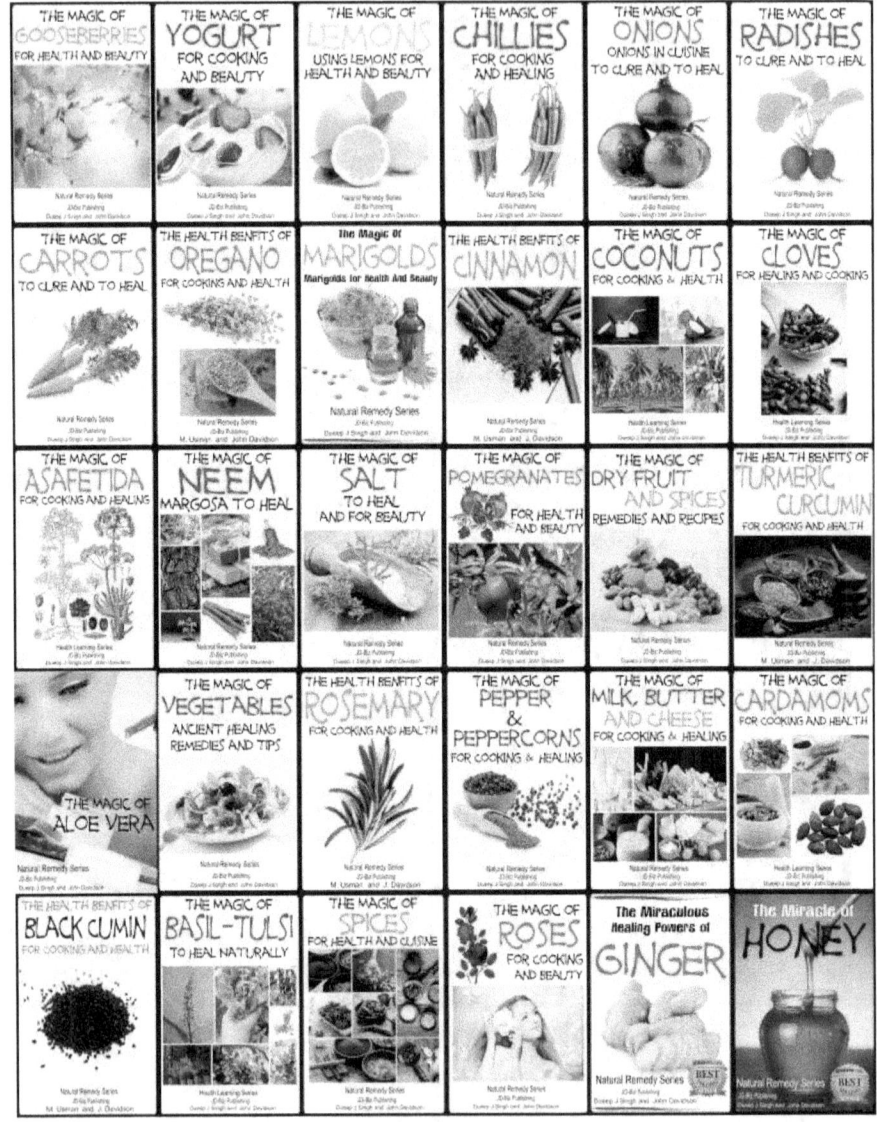

Country Life Books

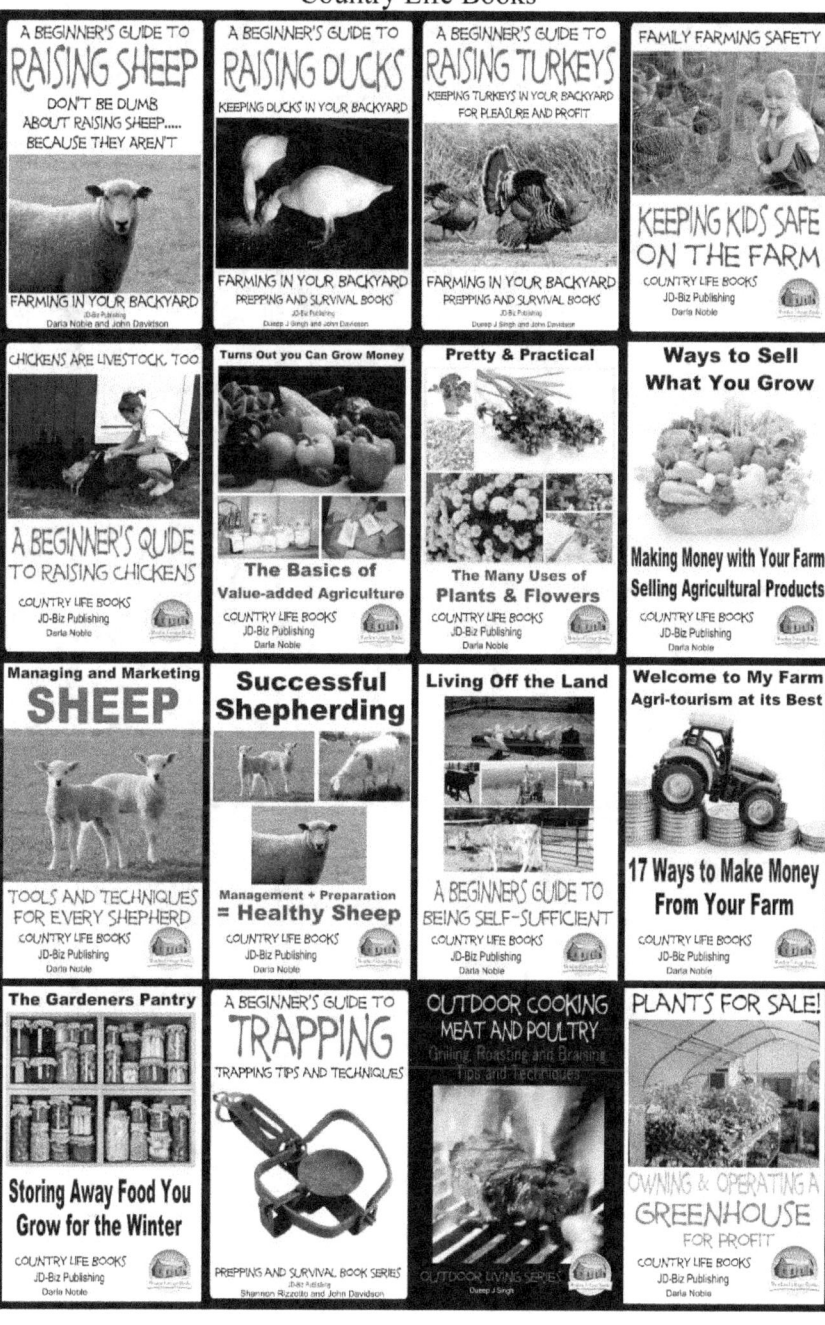

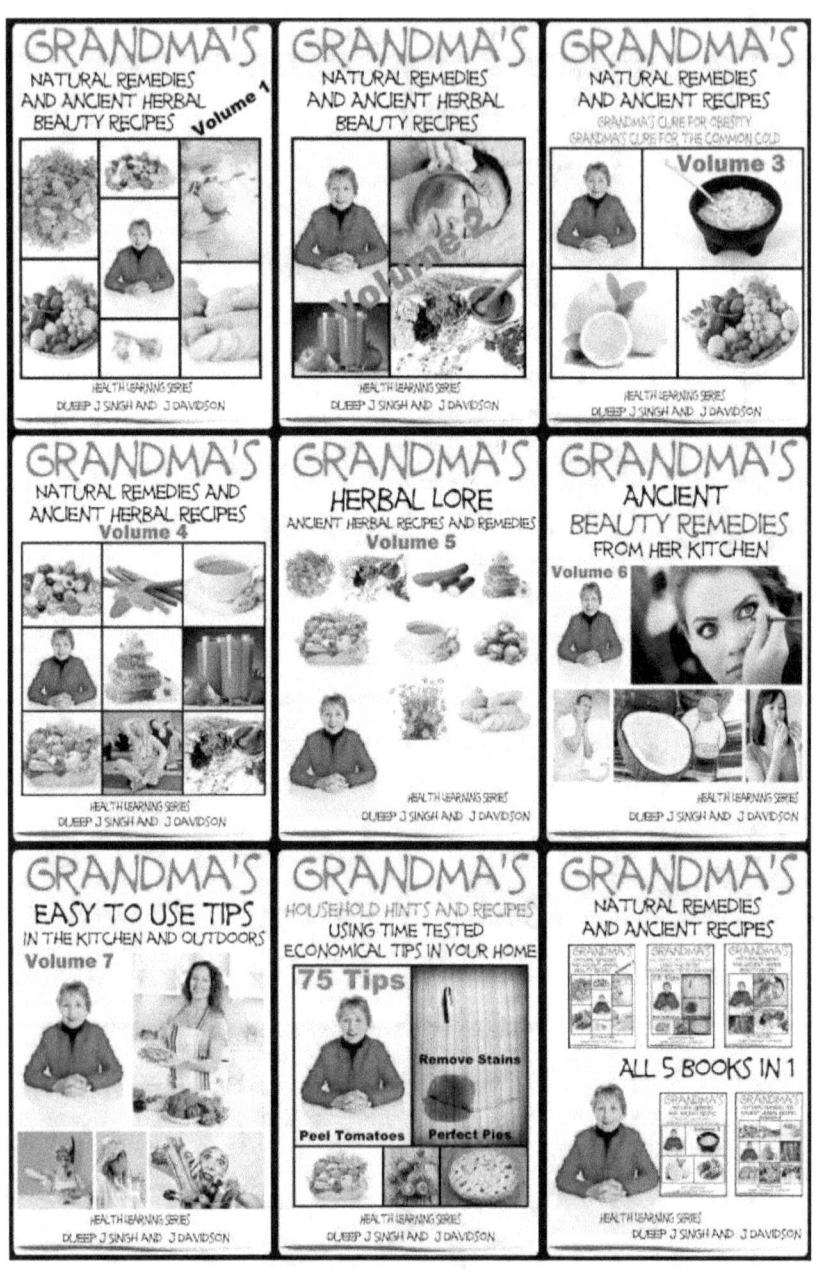

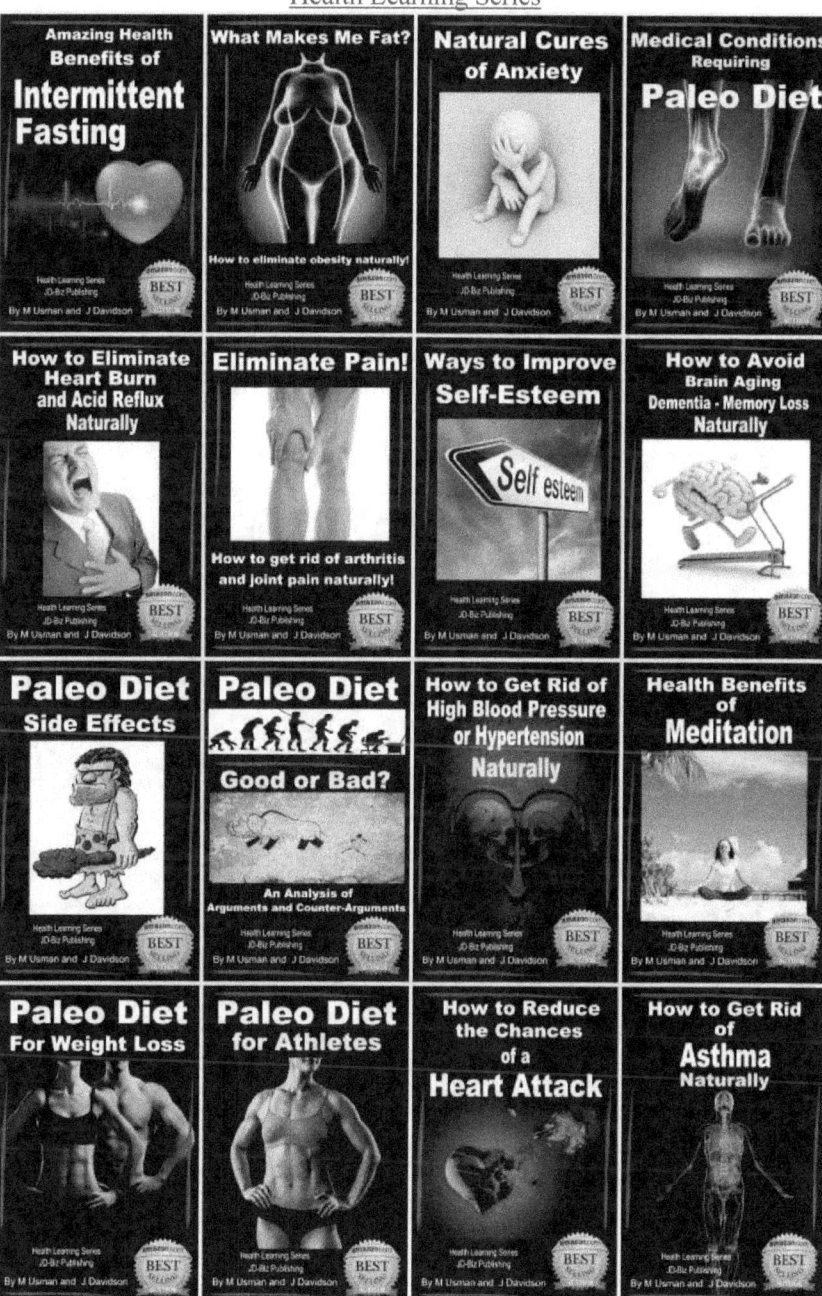

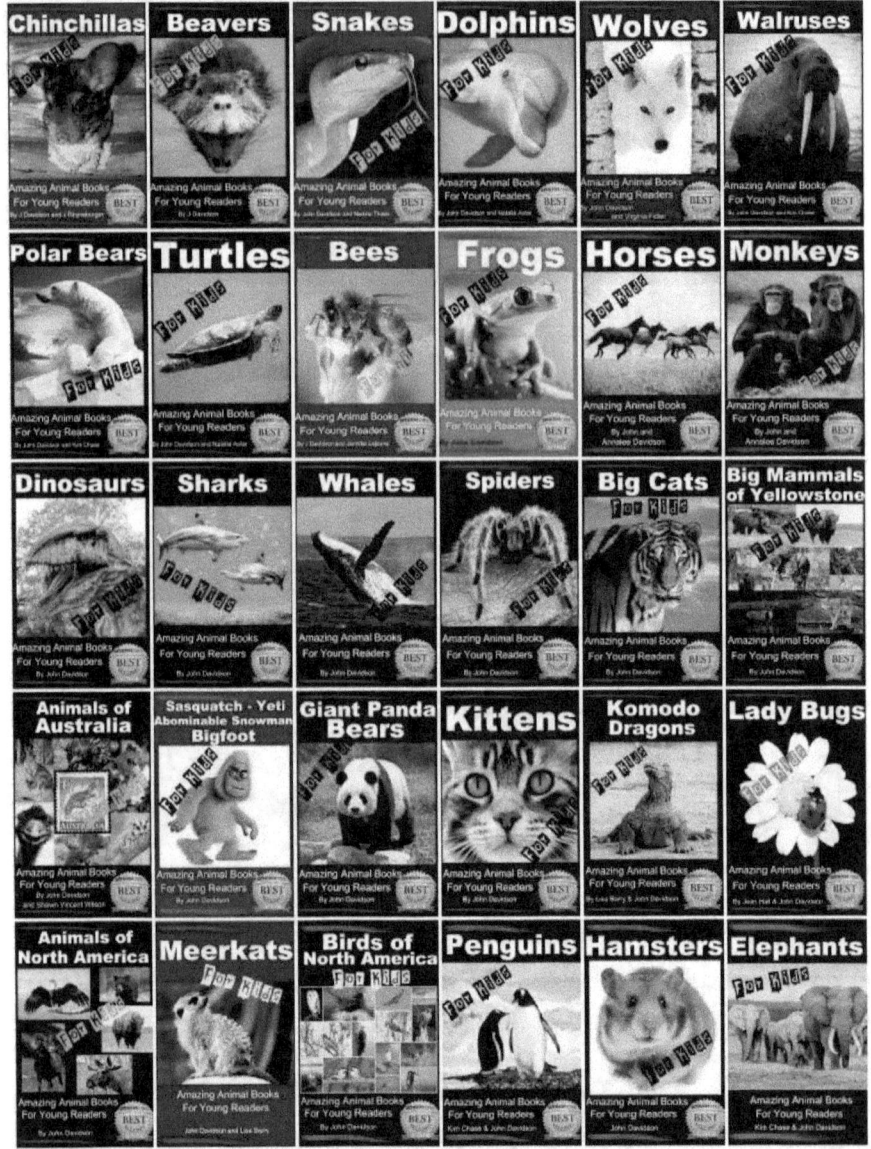

Learn To Draw Series

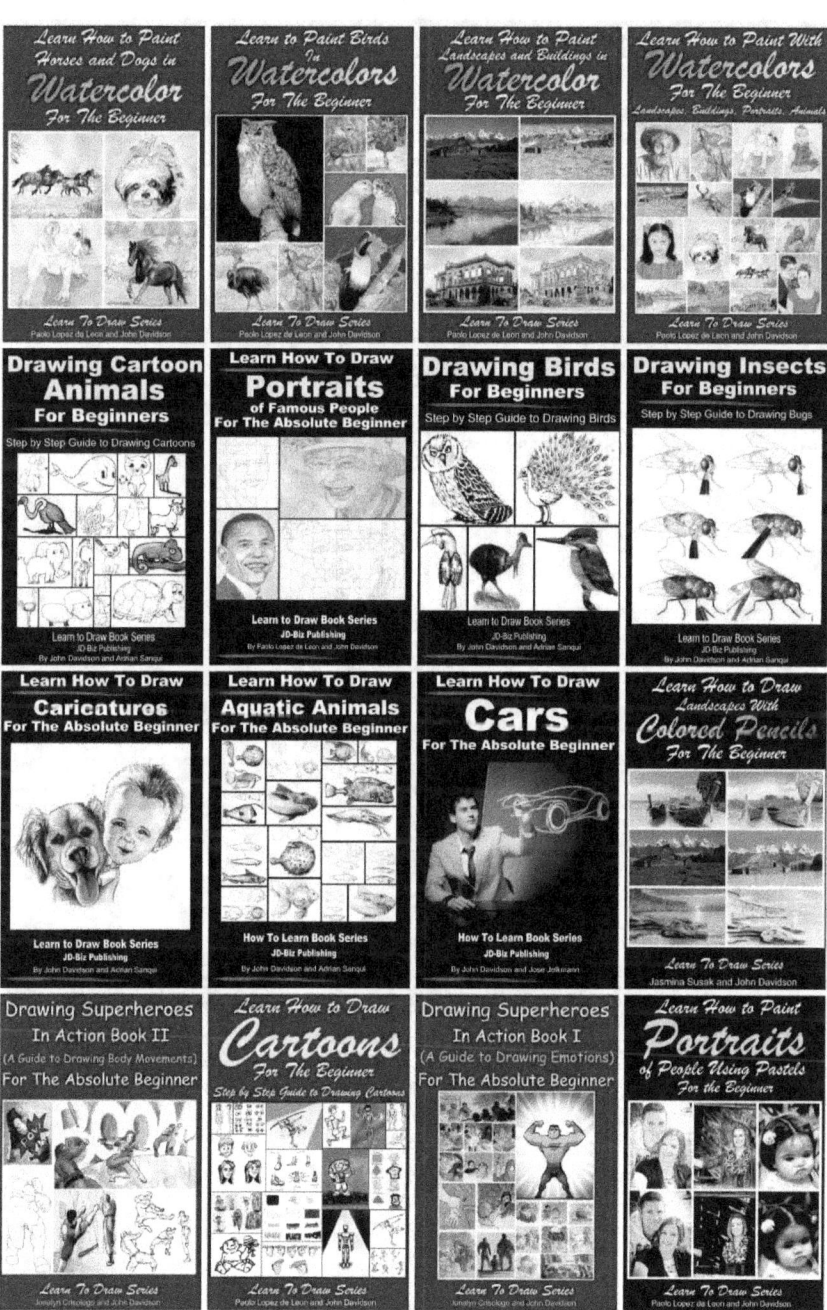

How to Build and Plan Books

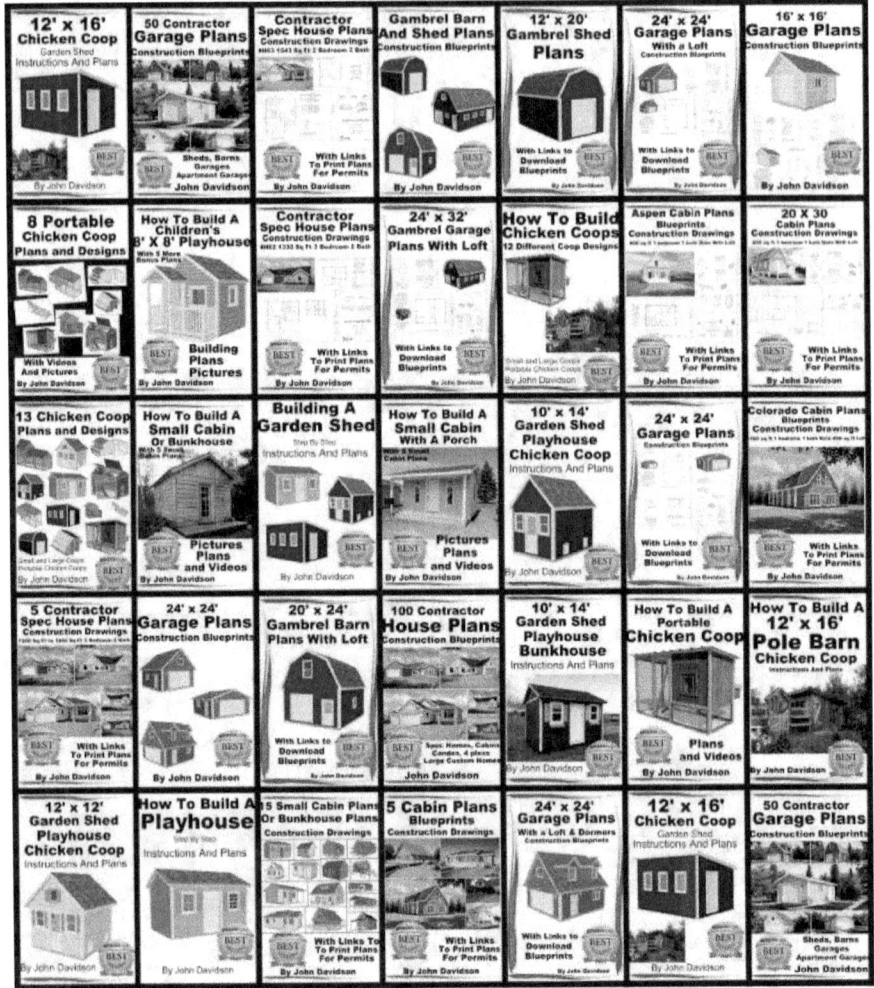

Entrepreneur Book Series

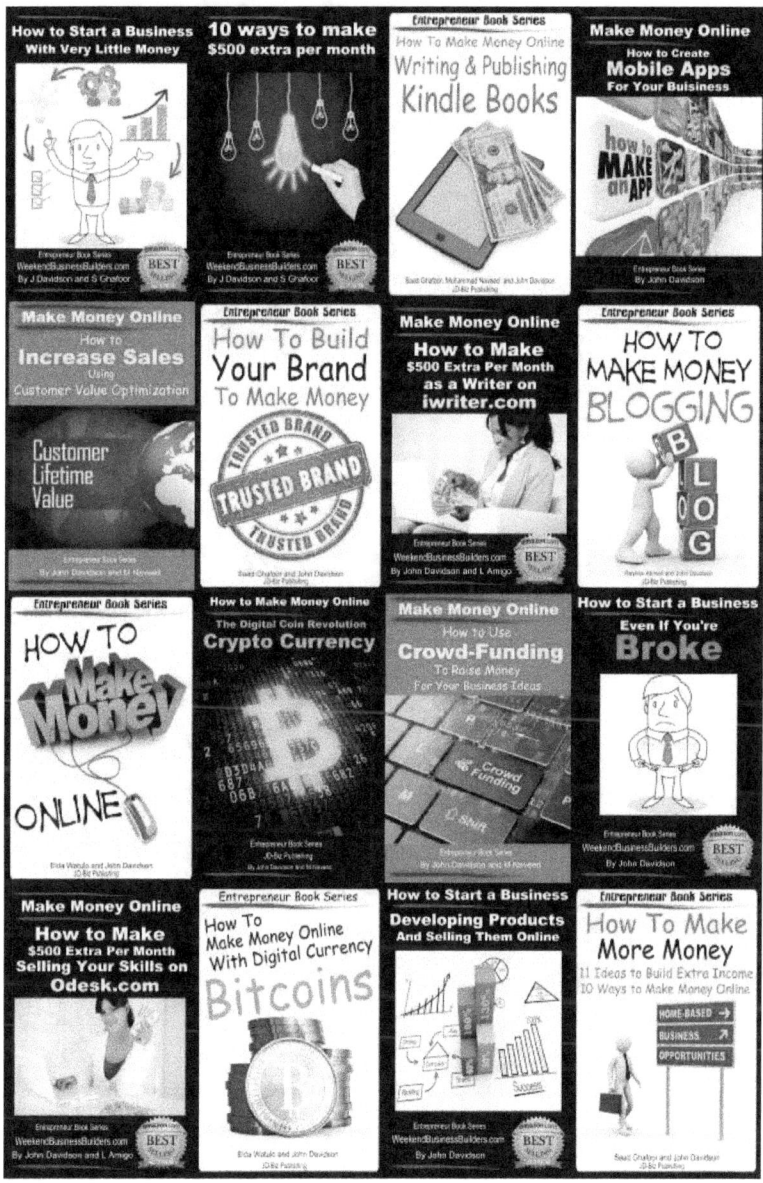

Our books are available at

1. Amazon.com

2. Barnes and Noble

3. Itunes

4. Kobo

5. Smashwords

6. Google Play Books

Download Free Books!

http://MendonCottageBooks.com

Publisher

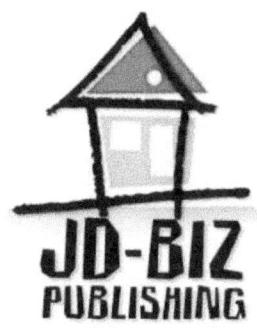

JD-Biz Corp

P O Box 374

Mendon, Utah 84325

http://www.jd-biz.com/

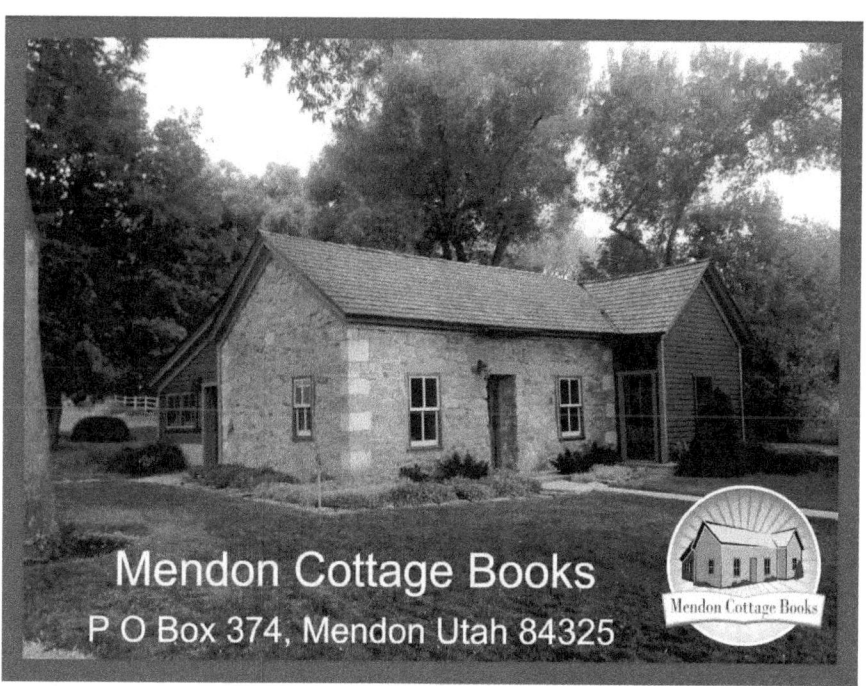

Mendon Cottage Books

P O Box 374, Mendon Utah 84325